COMMON SENSE

about

HEALTH CARE REFORM

in

AMERICA

by
John Geyman, M.D.

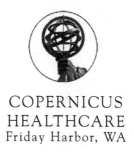

COPERNICUS
HEALTHCARE
Friday Harbor, WA

Common Sense About Health Care Reform in America

John Geyman, M.D.

Copernicus Healthcare
Friday Harbor, WA

First Edition

softcover: ISBN 978-1-938218-16-3

Library of Congress Control Number is
Available Upon Request From the Publisher

Copernicus Healthcare
34 Oak Hill Drive
Friday Harbor, WA 98250

www.copernicus-healthcare.org

Dedication

To the countless millions of Americans struggling under the cost and access burdens of our increasingly dysfunctional and unsustainable market-based health care system. May they and future generations finally have a system that works for all of us as its dedicated mission, not for the revenues of today's corporate profiteers.

NOTE TO THE READER

In his famous pamphlet, *Common Sense*, written for the people of the Thirteen Colonies in 1775-1776, Thomas Paine made a strong argument to gain independence from England. In clear and persuasive prose, he made a compelling case on moral and political grounds to fight for an egalitarian society and break from England. The pamphlet was widely sold to the 2.5 million people in the colonies, and was an instrumental force in energizing the American Revolution. Since then, it remains the all-time best selling title in American history, and is still in print today. In its early pages, under the heading of *Thoughts on the Present State of American Affairs*, Paine set out this goal 241 years ago:

> *In the following pages I offer nothing more than **simple facts**, **plain arguments**, and **common sense**; and have no other preliminaries to settle with the reader, than that he will divest himself from prejudice and prepossession, and suffer his reason and his feelings to determine for themselves . . . and generously enlarge his views beyond the present day.*

In the following pages written in 2017, I too offer simple facts, plain arguments, and common sense about health care in America.

Today, we have a crisis in U.S. health care with soaring costs and restricted access to health care in a highly bureaucratic, dysfunctional system dedicated to profits of corporate stakeholders, not the best interests of patients and their families. As the most expensive health care system in the world, we leave many millions of Americans out, resulting in higher numbers of preventable deaths and worse outcomes than other advanced countries around the world.

Previous attempts to reform our system have failed for more

1

than a century since Teddy Roosevelt's proposal for national health insurance in 1912. The economic and political power of corporate interests continue to block significant reform. To this day, we have neither addressed nor answered these three fundamental questions:

1. Is health care a right or a privilege based on ability to pay?

2. Who is the health care system for—patients and families or corporate stakeholders?

3. Is health care just another commodity for sale in a deregulated marketplace?

As a result, our government and we as taxpayers continue to bail out a failing private health insurance industry which will bankrupt us all unless we can break from the acquisitive tentacles of corporate interests.

Thus we now have a situation in health care parallel to that faced by Thomas Paine in the early days of this nation. We need to restructure our market-based health care system based on the needs of patients and families instead of the profits of corporate stakeholders in the medical-industrial complex. We need to face the facts of this crisis and broadly disseminate them to our population. We are now again involved in a bitter partisan debate over the future of health care. The corporate-owned mainstream media have largely failed to cover the substance of this debate, driven as they are by ratings and revenue for their own shareholders. After so many failed attempts over the years to reform our system, experience has shown that we must change how we finance health care in this country. We have three basic alternatives to do so— (1) continue, with revisions, the Affordable Care Act (ACA); (2) enact the Republican plan, the American Health Care Act (AHCA), or (3) adopt single-payer Medicare for All (H.R. 676 in the House of Representatives).

Where we go next will challenge our claimed democracy, but we can hope that evidence, experience, and an energized well informed electorate will finally bring universal access to health care as a human right in a just and sustainable system that is dedicated to the common good. Most advanced civilized countries around the world have achieved this many years ago. Today's political chaos may become our moment to do so, and I hope that this concise factual summary of the issues will help toward that goal.

A word about documentation of the facts described here—They are fully referenced in my recently released book, *Crisis in U.S. Health Care: Corporate Power vs. the Common Good*, which is reviewed on my website: johngeymanmd.org. For reasons of brevity, they are not listed herein.

I. COMPARISON OF THREE FINANCING ALTERNATIVES

Both the ACA and the Republican plan, the American Health Care Act (AHCA), are similar in retaining and continuing the government's bailout of the private health insurance industry. The third alternative—single-payer Medicare for All—would establish universal coverage to comprehensive health care for all Americans through a non-profit public financing system coupled with a private delivery system. It would ban private insurers from providing duplicate coverage to the public program, thereby eliminating our present multi-tier system.

These are the three basic alternatives facing us in trying to resolve today's system problems of restricted access, soaring costs and prices, growing unaffordability, and unacceptable quality of care for our population.

1. Continuation of the ACA with marginal improvements.

The ACA has brought significant improvements in access to care, including insuring 24 million Americans (especially through expansion of Medicaid in 31 states), requiring insurers to stop denying coverage for pre-existing conditions, and allowing parents to keep their children on their coverage until age 26. However, it falls short of our needs on many counts. There are still more than 28 million uninsured individuals with tens of millions more underinsured, and cost containment efforts have largely failed. The insurance market is now unstable and volatile, with some of the largest insurance giants threatening to leave entire markets for lack of sufficient profitability.

Proponents of improving the ACA propose bringing back the public option (dropped from consideration in 2009 due to opposition from the insurance industry), but this would have little chance of making much of a difference against the economic power and market share of private insurance giants. There would still be no mechanisms for containment of costs or prices. Other proposals would attempt to adjust ways in which insurers could be further protected from losses incurred by coverage of sicker patients, but these would just add to the coffers of insurers while further shifting costs of care to patients and taxpayers.

2. Repeal and replacement of the ACA by the AHCA (TrumpCare)

This has been a consistent goal of the GOP since the passage of the ACA in 2010, but the Republican Party has been unsuccessful in its repeal on some 60 occasions in the House. Since the 2016 elections, despite having control of the White House and both chambers of Congress, Republicans have been having great difficulty in coming up with a replacement plan that will pass, first in a divided House and then in the Senate. The provision of subsidies/tax credits, definition of essential health benefits, and cutbacks to Medicaid, have been especially controversial.

The first GOP plan for the AHCA was pulled from the House floor during President Trump's first 100 days when it became obvious that 24 million Americans would lose their health insurance and that there were not enough votes for its passage; public support for the bill was only 17 percent and President Trump's approval rating just 37 percent. Even corporate stakeholders in the present system, including the American Medical Association and American Hospital Association, came out against the bill as they faced the implications of smaller markets. Many GOP legislators faced angry crowds over health care in town halls across the country.

House Republicans then hastily drafted a revised bill, attempting to appease the hard right Freedom Caucus while gaining support from more moderate Republicans. The resulting bill includes these basic provisions:

- Eliminates the individual mandate and requirement for larger employers to offer employer-sponsored coverage.
- Allows states through waivers to limit essential health benefits.
- Reduces funding for Medicaid by $839 billion.
- Defunds Planned Parenthood.
- Replaces the ACA's subsidies with less generous tax credits.
- Allows insurers to charge seniors up to 5 times the rates for younger patients.
- Allows insurers to raise premiums on patients with pre-existing conditions, while providing (inadequate) funds for high-risk pools.

5

- Repeals taxes on pharmaceutical and medical device industries.
- Provides wealthy taxpayers $882 billion in tax breaks.

Without waiting for CBO scoring, the AHCA passed the House by a vote of 217 to 213 in early May, and was sent on to the Senate, where it is encountering formidable opposition in its present form. A 13-man working group in the Senate was charged with crafting its own bill, unfortunately without including any women in the group. Amidst this intense debate among congressional Republicans, it is unclear whether the Senate will ever pass a bill that can be passed in the House.

While the final details of a Republican replacement plan are not yet established, the main elements are likely to include such already discredited approaches as more cost-sharing with patients, health savings accounts (only higher-income individuals can afford them), selling insurance across state lines, high-risk pools, and deregulating the insurance industry. None of these approaches have been demonstrated to work in the past. High-risk pools, for example, have mostly collapsed due to inadequate funding. The case for the largest possible risk pool is made by one patient in Iowa with a complicated and serious genetic disorder receiving care costing $1 million a month, that recently forced the dominant insurer in the state's individual market to leave the state. (Hiltzik, M. *Los Angeles Times*, April 24, 2017) Such costs would virtually destroy a risk pool of 30,000 enrollees.

The AHCA would also stop open-ended funding for Medicaid, institute block grants to states, and allow states to cut back eligibility and benefit policies, thereby shredding an already porous safety net. Medicare and Medicaid would be further privatized.

3. Single-Payer Medicare for All (H.R. 676 in the House)

Based on the forgoing, this is our only **common sense** alternative to effectively reform U.S. health care. When enacted, all Americans will gain universal access to affordable, comprehensive health care regardless of their health status or income, with free choice of physician and hospital anywhere in the country. Benefits will include physician and hospital care, outpatient care, dental and vision services, rehabilitation, long-term care, mental health care, and prescription drugs. Medical bills will be generally eliminated, and there will be no co-payments or other out-of-pocket costs at the point of service. A single risk pool of 320 million Americans will spread risk effectively to accommodate the needs of the sickest patients, while saving enough money to assure universal access to care for everyone.

Table 1 compares multi-payer vs. single-payer financing of U.S. health care in terms of traditional American values.

TABLE 1

Alternative Financing Systems and American Values

TRADITIONAL VALUE	Single-Payer	Multi-Payer
Efficiency	↑	↓
Choice	↑	↓
Affordability	↑	↓
Actuarial value	↑	↓
Fiscal responsibility	↑	↓
Equitable	↑	↓
Accountable	↑	↓
Integrity	↑	↓
Sustainable	↑	↓

Source: Geyman, JP. *Health Care Wars: How Market Ideology and Corporate Power Are Killing Americans.* Friday Harbor, WA. Copernicus Healthcare, 2012, p. 198.

Table 2 compares the three basic reform alternatives:

(1) the Affordable Care Act (ACA), or ObamaCare,
(2) the GOP plan–the American Health Care Act (AHCA), or TrumpCare, and
(3) Single-Payer Medicare For All, or National Health Insurance (NHI).

TABLE 2

COMPARISON OF THREE REFORM ALTERNATIVES

	ACA	*GOP*	*NHI*
Access	Restricted	Restricted	Unrestricted
Choice	Restricted	Restricted	Unrestricted
Cost containment	No	No	Yes
Quality of care	Unimproved	Unimproved	Improved
Bureaucracy	Increased	Increased	Much reduced
Universal coverage	Never	Never	Immediately
Accountability	Limited	Limited	Yes
Sustainability	No	No	Yes

II. TODAY'S CRISIS IN HEALTH CARE

These are markers of **simple facts** that illustrate the depth and complexity of health care in America today.

Soaring costs of care

Despite the goal of the ACA to contain health care costs, they keep going up at uncontrolled rates seven years after it was enacted in 2010. In our system without significant price controls, individuals and families face increasing costs of insurance, higher deductibles, copayments, coinsurance, and out-of-pocket expenses. Even when insured, one-third of families receive additional surprise bills for out-of-network services they thought were covered. One in four Americans rank health care costs as their top concern, higher even above job security and unemployment.

Increasing unaffordability of care

The cost of health insurance and care for a typical family of four with an average employer-sponsored PPO health plan is now about $27,000 a year, having doubled over the last ten years (Milliman Medical Index, 2017). Many patients forgo or delay necessary care because of costs, resulting in worse outcomes later when and if they receive care. A one-year course of chemotherapy for cancer often ranges between $100,000 and $200,000, forcing many patients to choose between treatment and bankruptcy. More than seven in ten uninsured patients admitted to the hospital for trauma are at risk for catastrophic health care bills. Almost two million people go through bankruptcy every year because of medical bills and illness, despite most having had insurance, owning their own homes, having attended college, and having held responsible jobs.

Restricted access and choice of care

Except for evaluation and stabilization of emergencies in hospital ERs, access to health care depends largely on an individual's insurance status and ability to pay. Those with insurance are finding their choices of physicians and hospitals severely limited by insurers' narrowed networks, which can change with little notice from year to year. Many insurers have returned to the managed care era of the 1990s with built-in restrictions of choice that led to a strong consumer backlash then. Waiting times today can be lengthy even when physicians agree to see new patients, and many physicians refuse to see Medicaid patients.

Large numbers of uninsured and underinsured

Despite the ACA there are still more than 28 million uninsured Americans, including almost 5 million people in a "Medicaid coverage gap" in the 19 states that refused to expand Medicaid. Many states require Medicaid beneficiaries to pay premiums that force some patients to dis-enroll from these programs. Beyond the uninsured, there is a growing epidemic of underinsured people, whereby their health care costs exceed 10 percent of their annual household income. The Commonwealth Fund defines underinsurance as households spending 10 percent or more of their annual income on medical care (not including premiums) or 5 percent or more if their annual income is less than 200 percent of the federal poverty level. By these criteria, more than two of five underinsured adults cannot afford to seek needed care.

Inadequate primary care base

With the serious shortage of primary care physicians, it has become unusual for a patient and family to have and keep their own family doctor who knows them well over many years. Less than 10 percent of medical school graduates enter family medicine today, the broadest of the primary care specialties. The majority of internists and pediatricians leave primary care for subspecialties. This vacuum in primary care has led to the proliferation of urgent care centers for first-contact care, typically staffed by nurse practitioners and physician assistants, but without comprehensiveness, coordination, or continuity of care.

Disparities of care

Many groups in our population, especially people of color, face significant barriers and disparities in access to and utilization of health care, leading many to forgo necessary care and incur worse outcomes of care. There are many dimensions of disparities in health care, including race/ethnicity, socioeconomic status, age, gender, location, and disability status. These disparities result in a higher burden of illness, injury, disability, or mortality among disadvantaged groups. While the ACA made some improvements in this problem, disparities in care are still widespread across the U.S. They present an increasing challenge as the U.S. population becomes more diverse, with people of color projected to account for one-half of our population by 2045.

Unacceptable quality of care

We know that insurance coverage has much to do with access and quality of care that is received. The Centers for Disease Control and Prevention (CDC) estimated that 45,000 Americans died for lack of health insurance in 2012. Even when privately insured, one of three high-need patients have unmet needs, while the same number lack dental insurance. Overutilization of care is also a problem, since it is estimated that one third of all health care services provided are unnecessary, inappropriate, and often even harmful. The U.S. consistently ranks poorly among 11 advanced countries studied by the Commonwealth Fund, as illustrated in the 2014 rankings: #11 in overall ranking, cost-restricted access, efficiency, equity, and healthy lives.

Marginalization and criminalization of mental illness

Stigma of mental disorders has long been a problem in the U.S., with mental health care not receiving parity by payers with physical illness. Many state mental hospitals have been closed over the years, resulting in many patients with severe mental illness being held in emergency rooms, hospitals, and jails ("psychiatric boarding") without treatment as they await a bed, sometimes for weeks. A 2016 report by Mental Health America found that more than one-half of these patients receive insufficient treatment or none at all. Psychiatric and behavioral problems among minority youth often lead to in school punishment or incarceration, but rarely mental health care.

Inadequate safety net

Although the ACA expanded funding for community health centers, we still have a very porous safety net that fails the needs of many Americans, especially the uninsured and underinsured. Many physicians will not see Medicaid patients because of low reimbursement. States vary widely in their eligibility and benefit policies, with many restrictive to the extreme. This problem is likely to become much worse if and when the current Republican Congress and administration implement block grants to the states, with decreased federal involvement.

Decline of physicians' clinical autonomy and increasing burnout

With almost two-thirds of U.S. physicians employed by large corporate groups, especially expanding hospital systems, they are under pressure to be "more productive" in terms of generating more revenue for their employers. This boils down to seeing more patients in a shorter period of time, ordering more tests and procedures, and dealing with the huge bureaucracy of our multi-payer insurance system. A 2016 study found that more than one-half of U.S. physicians spend more than 10 hours each week on paperwork, while a 2014 study showed that family physicians and internists were spending 17 hours a week on these tasks. About one-half of family physicians and internists are experiencing burnout. Many are considering early retirement, with the most common complaint being the burden of "too many bureaucratic tasks" and their frustration with reduced face-to-face time with their patients.

Massive, inefficient bureaucracy

With some 1,300 private health insurers in our multi-payer financing system, the U.S. is by far the most expensive system in the world. The overhead of the private insurance industry now amounts to $792 per capita, more than five times that of Canada with its single-payer public financing system. Hospital administrative costs in the U.S. account for more than 25 percent of total hospital expenditures, while administrators in various parts of the system have grown by 3,000 percent since 1970. Nurses in this country spend more than 13 hours per week to obtain prior authorizations for services, compared to none in Canada.

III. SOME HISTORICAL PERSPECTIVE

Corporatization and consolidation have transformed U.S. health care from a cottage industry in the 1960s to an enormous medical-industrial complex today. Much of this transformation has taken place since the 1980s as part of the neoconservative movement. While theorists in market theory tout the belief that increased market power brings economies of scale that will contain costs and add to value for consumers, that theory has proven to be a myth in health care.

Another myth disproven by experience over the last three decades is that the private sector is more efficient than the public sector. Hence the trend toward privatization of public programs like Medicare and Medicaid as well as increasing privatization of entire parts of the health care system. Figure 1 shows the remarkable degree to which parts of our health care system are now privatized in for-profit ownership.

FIGURE 1

EXTENT OF FOR-PROFIT OWNERSHIP, 2016

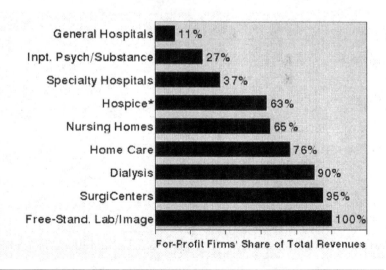

General Hospitals	11%
Inpt. Psych/Substance	27%
Specialty Hospitals	37%
Hospice*	63%
Nursing Homes	65%
Home Care	76%
Dialysis	90%
SurgiCenters	95%
Free-Stand. Lab/Image	100%

For-Profit Firms' Share of Total Revenues

Source: Commerce Department, Service Annual Survey 2016 or most recent available data for share of establishments.

13

The emphasis on short-term profits for CEOs and shareholders has replaced the traditional service ethic of earlier years with a profit-driven business "ethic," with lack of accountability to the public interest. As one example of this transformation, private Medicare HMO insurers, in pursuit of their business model, soon became expert at marketing their plans to healthier people, avoiding sicker enrollees, and cherry picking the market through favorable risk selection, all the while seeking protection from the government for any losses.

Another major change over the last 50 years has been the exponential growth in specialization and sub-specialization. There are now some 150 member boards and certified sub-specialties listed by the American Board of Medical Specialties. Since that trend has been associated with a major decline of primary care, we now have a serious shortage of primary care physicians. As a result, the average patient has multiple physicians, each for a different health problem, with increased fragmentation and loss of continuity of care. Medical school graduates, with debts at time of graduation typically in the $100,000 to $200,000 range, avoid primary care and seek out such higher paying specialties as radiology, orthopedic surgery, anesthesiology, and dermatology. Another major trend has been the separation of outpatient care from hospital care. Hospitalists now coordinate inpatient care, which is increasingly fragmented among specialties and even among hospitalists themselves.

I am indebted to Dr. Donald Frey, professor of family medicine at Creighton University in Omaha, Nebraska, for this graphic that gives us an overall picture of U.S. health care today.

FIGURE 2

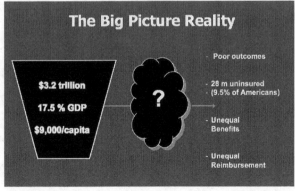

IV. LESSONS FROM PREVIOUS REFORM FAILURES

These are some of the main takeaway lessons as **plain arguments** that we should learn from the U.S. experience with market-based health care over the last 40 years.

1. Market failure

We can't avoid knowing that health care markets do not work like other markets in our economy, where competition can keep prices and costs down and consumers can shop for the best deal. Instead, consolidation among corporate stakeholders has led to increasing prices, whether in the insurance, hospital, drug or medical device industries. Moreover, patients typically can't predict or know their needs, urgency of time is often a factor in their decision-making, and comparative information is neither transparent nor available. Patients, physicians, and insurers are all dealing with uncertainty.

2. Consumer directed health care (CDHC) has failed to control health care spending.

This concept—that "empowered patients with more skin in the game" will contain health care costs by being more judicious in seeking care—has been completely discredited over the last three decades. However, it remains an underlying principle of private health insurers as they impose higher deductibles, co-payments, coinsurance and other restrictions on enrollees. It is now well known that increased cost sharing with patients leads them to forgo or delay necessary care and incur worse outcomes. This is a mechanism by which employers, insurers, and federal/state governments can shift more responsibility from themselves to patients and their families.

3. The private health insurance industry is obsolete and should be abandoned.

This industry has had a long run, but is antithetical to reform as it continues to game the system for higher revenues for its CEOs and shareholders at the expense of patients and taxpayers.

The ACA has been generous to private insurers, allowing them to still find ways to discriminate against the sick by such means as high cost-sharing, inadequate provider networks, restrictive drug formularies, and deceptive marketing practices. Even while receiving large subsidies from the government, it consumes 15 to 20 percent of the health care dollar in bureaucracy, administrative overhead, and profits as it retains a top position on Wall Street's S&P 500. Its financial success is still based on segmenting the risk pool in its favor and avoiding sicker patients if possible. The ACA bailed the industry out seven years ago, as both ACA defenders and proponents of a Republican plan in Congress hope to do once again today. But even CEOs of some insurers acknowledge that the industry is in a "death spiral" as its products become more unaffordable and offer less coverage. Many insurers are predicting large premium increases in 2018, even as many leave markets that they deem insufficiently profitable.

4. Deregulated health care markets fail the common good.

Although we are being assured constantly that less regulation will somehow foster more competition in health care, long experience shows that this is a myth. Two examples make the point.

- Under the ACA, for example, regulation of insurers has been lax. Most regulatory authority has been handed over to the states, where insurance lobbyists dominate state capitols. As a result, control of premiums has been generous to insurers, as have requirements for provider networks, and insurers have been able to avoid a federal requirement to report executive and employee compensation data. According to the Center for Public Integrity, one-half of state insurance commissioners who left their jobs in the last ten years went to work for the industry they were supposed to be regulating. An April 2017 final rule by CMS further accommodates insurers by shortening their annual open enrollment periods, giving them more flexibility to offer plans of less value at lower premiums and higher deductibles, and end federal review of network adequacy.

- The drug industry has successfully lobbied for lax regulation for many years through its trade organization, PhRMA. It has avoided importation of drugs from Canada and other countries, while resisting negotiated drug prices as the Veterans Administration has effectively done for many years. Under the recently enacted 21st Century Cures Act, standards for FDA approval of new drugs have been drastically lowered, so that rigorous random-controlled trials are no longer required for approval, just "real world evidence" shown by uncontrolled observational data collected by the drug companies themselves.

5. Privatization doesn't work; it is inefficient and gouges us for profits.

There continues to be a prevailing myth, promoted by market enthusiasts, that the private sector is more efficient than public programs. Medicare gives us a good example that completely rebuts that myth. Conceived and enacted in 1965 as a social insurance program because of the failure of the private sector to meet the needs of older Americans, traditional Medicare offered for the first time a comprehensive set of health care benefits to all people age 65 and older. It represented seven values and public policy concerns: *financial security, equity, efficiency, affordability over time, political accountability, political sustainability,* and *maximizing individual liberty.* Since then, it has proven to be a solid rock in an increasingly volatile health care marketplace, and has been run with a low administrative overhead of about 2.5 percent.

Over the succeeding years, especially since the 1990s, there has been a strong effort by private insurers to privatize Medicare, and more recently Medicaid, as they tell us that they offer more value and choice. Instead, they operate with administrative costs five times higher that traditional Medicare, cherry pick the market for favorable risk selection, and dis-enroll sicker people, all the while receiving many billions of overpayments from the government ($283 billion between 1985 and 2008). Here again, they withdraw from the market if not sufficiently profitable. Table 3 compares privatized Medicare with traditional public Medicare.

TABLE 3

Comparative Features of Privatized and Public Medicare

PRIVATIZED MEDICARE	ORIGINAL MEDICARE
Experience-rated eligibility	Universal coverage
Managed competition	Social insurance as earned right
Defined contribution	Defined benefits
Segmented risk pool	Broad risk pool
Market pricing to risk	Administered prices
More volatile access & benefits	More reliable access & benefits
Increased cost sharing	Less cost sharing
Less accountability	Potential for more accountability
Less choice of provider & hospital	Full choice of provider & hospital
Less well distributed	Well distributed
Less efficiency, higher overhead	More efficiency, lower overhead

Source: Geyman, JP. *Shredding the Social Contract The Privatization of Medicare.* Monroe, ME. *Common Courage Press,* 2006, p.206

Today, about one-third of Medicare beneficiaries are in private Medicare plans, as well as more than one-half of 66 million people enrolled in Medicaid. The government has been subsidizing these programs for a very long time. In fact, almost two-thirds of our supposedly private health care system is now paid for by the government—with our taxes!

6. Health care is not just another commodity for sale in an open market, but an essential human right.
    The U.S. still stands alone as an outlier among most advanced countries around the world in not accepting health care as a basic human right. The dominant culture of our market-based system treats health care services as commodities in an open market with access a privilege based on ability to pay. It is all about money in a multi-tiered system based on our income levels. Corpo-

rate stakeholders in our medical-industrial complex see health care as a large industry with opportunities for their financial bottom lines to drive policy and access to care. This approach disregards the fact that we are all in the same boat—regardless of our incomes. We will all have some or many times in our lives when an accident or serious illness will diminish our futures or even force us into bankruptcy. As health insurance and care exceed the budgets of more and more of our population, it becomes increasingly clear that our system is unfair, inhumane, cruel, and inadequate.

7. Today's market-based health care system is falling apart and is not sustainable without fundamental financing reform.

We have yet to accept that accommodating the self-interests of corporate stakeholders in our for-profit market-based system will never give us cost containment and affordable access to care for our population. Politicians and legislators in the past have succumbed to industry's massive lobbying campaign, buying them off in both major political parties. Meeting their self-interest just leads to more profiteering and gaming the market on the backs of patients, their families, and taxpayers. We need financing reform that gets rid of our huge bureaucratic and wasteful multi-payer system. Remember the three questions, still unanswered, that we started with:

1. Is health care a right or a privilege based on ability to pay?

2. Who is the health care system for— patients and families or corporate stakeholders?

3. Is health care just another commodity for sale in a deregulated marketplace?

Real health care reform must answer these questions before setting out on just one more unfair, overly expensive system that fails the public interest. With the government paying for almost two-thirds of the costs of health care, there is already plenty of money in the system if we cut the profiteering and waste and redirect it to universal access to affordable health care for all Americans.

8. We need a larger role of government to reform the system.

Instead of the neoconservative agenda of past, recent and current administrations that promote budget cutting, less government, further deregulation, shifting responsibility for federal programs to the states, and trickle down economics with corporate tax cuts, we need a larger and more accountable and efficient role of government acting in the public interest. Recent decades have proven that corporate interests of the medical-industrial complex will never give us a sustainable system that meets the health care needs of all Americans. Whether we realize it or not, we are approaching a breaking point that now requires fundamental financing reform.

John Adams, second president of the United States and one of our founding fathers, had it right about the role of government:

> *Government is instituted for the common good: for the protection, safety, prosperity and happiness of the people; and not for the profit, honor, or private interest of any one man, family or class of men.*

Jacob B Hacker, Ph.D., professor of political science at Yale University and co-author of the 2016 book, *American Amnesia: How the War on Government Led Us to Forget What Made America Prosper*, recently made this useful observation:

> *The difference between the United States and other countries isn't the role of insurance; it's the role of government. More specifically, it's the way in which those who benefit from America's dysfunctional market have mobilized to use government to protect their earnings and profits. . . . But in every other rich country, the government not only provides coverage to all citizens; it also provides strong counter pressure to those who seek to use their inherent market power to raise prices or deliver lucrative but unnecessary services . . .*

(Hacker, JB, Why an open market won't repair American health care. *New York Times*, April 4, 2017)

V. HOW MEDICARE FOR ALL WILL WORK

Medicare for All will be national health insurance (NHI) on a **common sense** basis similar to that of many other advanced countries around the world. Patients have only to present their NHI card when seeking care, and the administrative overhead of the new system will be cut by about five-fold. Costs can be contained through a large risk pool, negotiated annual budgets with hospitals and other facilities, negotiated fees with physicians, and negotiated drug prices through bulk purchasing (as the VA has done for years). We will save about $616 billion a year as soon as NHI is implemented ($503 billion by eliminating administrative overhead and $113 billion on outpatient prescription drugs). These savings will be redirected to patient care through a more efficient system that can pay for universal coverage of our entire population.

Health professionals will still have their own private practices while hospitals, nursing homes and other facilities will not be owned by the government—so this will not be socialized medicine. Provisions will be made to transition private for-profit facilities over to not-for-profit status during a transition period of about 15 years. Funds will also be provided for re-training of many people working in various capacities in the present system.

Most will win under NHI. Patients, families and taxpayers will receive much more than they do now for less money. Employers will be relieved of their burden to provide health insurance to their employees, while gaining a healthier workforce and becoming more competitive in the global economy. Federal and state governments will save money with simpler administration in a service-oriented system no longer driven by bottom-line revenues to corporate interests. Physicians and other providers, freed from paperwork and bureaucracy, will have more time for direct patient care. The big loser, of course, will be the private insurance industry, but it has not demonstrated enough accountability and value to patients and society to be further bailed out by taxpayers.

NHI will be funded by a progressive funding plan. As examples, those with incomes of $50,000 pay $1,500 in taxes, increasing to $6,000 for those with incomes about $100,000 and $12,000 for those with incomes of $200,000. Ninety-five percent of Americans will pay less than they do now for insurance and care. That will be a huge change from our current bills for health insurance and care, which now average more than $25,000 a year for a typical family of four with an average Preferred Provider Organization (PPO) in an employer-sponsored plan.

Table 4 shows how single-payer NHI will improve the quality of health care for all Americans, as conceptualized by Dr. Gordon Schiff, associate professor of internal medicine at Harvard Medical School.

Table 4
How Single-Payer NHI Will Improve Quality of Care

Access	• Everyone automatically eligible/ensured access; only plan for true universal insurance and access. • Able to control cost globally (w/ fences) so no reliance on access barriers to maintain affordability.
User-Friendly Simple	• A "no depends" system-no complicated rules, exchanges, variations by age, state, income, disease, employment/employer, marital status, etc. • Avoids eligibility determinations, means testing,confusion, enrollment complexities.
Single Standard	• By definition single system with fair rules for all • Generates database to identify disparities and track effectiveness of interventions
Continuity	• No switching for change in employment, divorce, new private insurance plan, restricted networks • Ensured reimbursement permitting provider financial stability.
Choice	• Avoids negative features and restricted networks, choice of provider and hospitals. • Uniform reimbursement and benefits package enables portability and ability to choose
Nursing	• Stable source of funding for hospitals via global budgets • Potentials for national standards, support for nursing education, less frustrations with arbitrary financially-driven anti-nurse cost cutting
Time	• All patients would be covered; ensuring provider is reimbursed for his/her time w/ each. • Greater potential for support of teamwork resulting from continuities of patients, staff, funding
Caring Commitment	• Elimination of greed, profit, corporate controls as the drivers health care system decision making • Restoring ability of professionals to advocate for patients and a better system, rather than current structured antagonisms
Clinical Information Systems	• Role and necessity of national standards, federal leadership in funding IT, demonstrated VA leadership, other countries lead • Design for clinical needs of patients, providers, not insurers, vendors (accountablity w/ unified system) • Ability to collect and aggregate data for quality oversight
Communication	• Better positioned to overcome trade secrets/secrecy inherent in private control • In avoiding financial barriers for patients to seek care, call, lower threshold/barriers for communication.
Continuous Improvement	• Stable public systems, "in business of health" for the long haul thus ROI on quality investment • Noteworthy successes of CQI in public sector (VA,Navy)
Accountability	• Public system by definition public & accountable, especially if democratic decision-making, organized advocacy efforts, vigilant media scrutiny, • Role that Medicare, Medicaid (and hence public insurance data) has played in outcomes evaluation and review of allocation decisions.
Prevention Oriented	• Unlike private plans where prevention does not pay due to frequent patient switches, greater incentives for prevention • Public system can be best integrated with public health at local and national levels

VI. HOW WE CAN MAKE IT HAPPEN

Whatever Congress and the Republican administration does about repealing/replacing the ACA or failing that, sabotaging it through administrative actions by Dr. Tom Price, the new head of the Department of Health Care and Human Services (DHHS), Republicans will own and take the blame for the new chaotic market-based system. There is already clear evidence that the political stakes and dynamics are changing markedly as the GOP confronts the backlash from people facing loss of their health insurance and the lack of public support for GOP proposals. Trump Care will disappoint his original supporters when they see that it makes his rhetoric of "a wonderful system that will take care of everyone" just another empty promise.

Since the GOP plan also allows insurers to charge seniors up to five times as much as younger enrollees, seniors and the AARP are mobilizing against that proposal. Possible inclusion of defunding of Planned Parenthood, as well as insurers charging women more than men for insurance, increases women's resistance to the GOP plan.

Increasing market uncertainty throughout health care markets also sends new fears of threats to future markets for other parts of the medical-industrial complex, including hospitals (especially in rural areas), pharmaceutical and medical device companies. As the numbers of uninsured and underinsured grow, consumers will be even more unable to afford care.

Gaining momentum since the withdrawal of the AHCA from a House vote, Medicare for All (H. R. 676) has gained 110 co-sponsors in the House, Senator Bernie Sanders plans to bring forward a similar bill in the Senate, and public polls show a growing majority of support for universal health care as well as a larger role of government to assure this care. Surprisingly, a May 2016 Gallup poll found that 41 percent of Republicans and leaners favored replacing the ACA with Medicare for All. Another 2016 poll of small business owners in California, for the first time in years of surveys, found that a majority supported Medicare for All. As Eugene Robinson observed in a recent editorial: "With their anti-Obamacare fanaticism, Republicans are putting single-payer on the table." (Robinson, E. Republicans are accidentally paving the way for single payer health care. *Washington Post*, May 8, 2017)

A growing number of professional organizations have become proactive in working toward universal health care, including Physicians for a National Health Program (PNHP) with 22,000 members in all specialties, the American College of Physicians, the American Psychiatric Association, and the American Society of Clinical Oncology, and the American Nursing Association. Although the American Medical Association has long opposed any such system, Dr. Howard Bauchner, Editor in Chief of *The Journal of the American Medical Association*, recently stated:

> *All physicians, including those who are members of Congress, other health professionals, and professional societies (should) speak with a single voice and say that health care is a basic right for every person, and not a privilege to be available and affordable only for a majority.*

Today's chaotic and dysfunctional system can be fixed, but only through fundamental financing reform, which is required sooner than later. We need to build on a growing anti-Trump movement of resistance, and insistence for Medicare for All.

Powerful corporate stakeholders and many Republican politicians stand in the way of real reform. In addition, the "mainstream" media, owned as they are by large corporate interests, have to be held accountable for investigative and objective reporting of developments in the struggle for universal health care. Indivisible, created by former congressional staffers who observed and learned from the rapid political success of the Tea Party, outline in their *Practical Guide for Resisting the Trump Agenda* concrete ways in which the broad public can become activists for this kind of change wherever they live.

In these political times, it may well be that Democrats, if they take a more progressive and leadership stance, can take back the House in the 2018 elections. The next several years may well bring the moment to adopt a national health program that meets the needs of all Americans, not just the corporate few.

We can be inspired toward that goal by these two health policy experts and champions of social justice:

Forget trying to tweak AHCA by placing conservative principles above patient service. Also forget trying to tweak ACA by placing the concepts of incrementalism and supposed political feasibility above patient service. Let's go for the model that places patients first—a well designed, single-payer national health program—an improved Medicare for All.

—Dr. Don McCanne, retired family physician, Senior Health Policy Fellow and former president of Physicians for a National Health Program

From my adolescent years to the present, I've never wavered in my belief in humanity's ability—and our collective responsibility—to bring about a more just and equitable social order. I've always believed in humanity's potential to create a more caring society . . . The future can be bright, but only if we work to make it so.

—The late Dr. Quentin Young, internist, long-time activist toward social justice in health care, and author of the 2013 book, *Everybody In Nobody Out: Memoirs of a Rebel Without a Pause*

ABOUT THE AUTHOR

John Geyman, M.D. is professor emeritus of family medicine at the University of Washington School of Medicine in Seattle, where he served as Chairman of the Department of Family Medicine from 1976 to 1990. As a family physician with over 21 years in academic medicine, he also practiced in rural communities for 13 years. He was the founding editor of *The Journal of Family Practice* (1973 to 1990) and the editor of 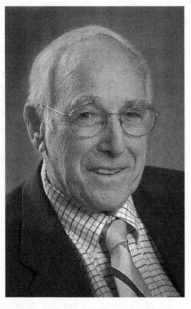 *The Journal of the American Board of Family Medicine* from 1990 to 2003. Since 1990 he has been involved with research and writing on health policy and health care reform. He served as president of Physicians for a National Health Program from 2005 to 2007, and is a member of the National Academy of Medicine.

His books include:

Crisis in U.S Health Care: Corporate Power vs. the Common Good (2017)

The Human Face of ObamaCare: Promises vs. Reality and What Comes Next (2016)

How ObamaCare is Unsustainable: Why We Need a Single-Payer Solution for All Americans (2015)

Souls on a Walk: An Enduring Love Story Unbroken by Alzheimer's (2012)

Health Care Wars: How Market Ideology and Corporate Power Are Killing Americans (2012)

Breaking Point: How the Primary Care Crisis Endangers the Lives of Americans. (2011)

Hijacked: The Road to Single-Payer in the Aftermath of Stolen Health Care Reform (2010)

The Cancer Generation: Baby Boomers Facing a Perfect Storm (2009)

Do Not Resuscitate: Why the Health Insurance Industry is Dying, and How We Must Replace It (2008)

The Corrosion of Medicine: Can the Profession Reclaim Its Moral Legacy? (2008)

Shredding the Social Contract: The Privatization of Medicare (2006)

Falling Through the Safety Net: Americans Without Health Insurance (2005)

The Corporate Transformation of Health Care: Can the Public Interest Still Be Served? (2004)

Health Care in America: Can Our Ailing System Be Healed? (2002)

Family Practice: Foundation of Changing Health Care (1985)

The Modern Family Doctor and Changing Medical Practice (1971)

Copies can be ordered for $5.95 per copy
from Amazon.com and CreateSpace.com

Made in the USA
Middletown, DE
08 July 2017